NCLEX PN
100 Pharmacology Questions with Rationales

Copyright 2016 Nursing Aids

INTRODUCTION

Pharmacology is one of the most challenging subjects in nursing, not only because there is over a thousand drugs out there in the market to be familiar with, but also because pharmacology is a part of every aspect of patient care. In fact, it is a hefty part of medical-surgical nursing, pediatrics, maternal and child, geriatrics, hospice, psychiatric nursing and even community nursing. When flipping through the pages of a 3-inch thick drug handbook, would-be nurses feel a great sense of frustration. They ask themselves, *"How do I study this?", "Which information should I focus on?"*.

A proven strategy in becoming successful in Pharmacology is familiarizing oneself with the drugs. One way of doing this is to answer as many NCLEX-style questions on Pharmacology as you can and then study their rationales. This narrows down concepts to the most significant ones. Another strategy is to look at concepts that deal with safety issues. Many questions revolve around safety. It is the primary concern in Pharmacology. Have there been new drugs introduced in the last 3-5 years? Zero-in on that, too. Do research on certain issues that actually happened in real life that greatly affected patient outcomes.

These strategies are going to work wonders in achieving your goals in becoming a registered nurse, but to dig into books just to look for concepts that deal with safety, and doing research on true-to-life accounts are too time consuming.

This is the main reason why you need this 100-question book. The reliability of this book is ensured because nursing instructors who are experts in the field of Pharmacology developed the questions themselves. Its purpose is to serve as a very useful tool in familiarizing aspiring nurses with the concepts. More importantly, it gives a fair head start in the NCLEX review because the instructors have done the digging and the research part for you!

Here in this book, you will have a compilation of questions that revolve around safety and positive patient outcomes. It will also feature new approved drugs and the concerns in their use. It will also include current topics on Pharmacology, with up-to-date information that will most likely come out in the NCLEX examination. It will give you the right concepts, and it will save you time especially during the hectic days of NCLEX preparation. So get your head start now!

1. The nurse is caring for several patients who are on intravenous antibiotic therapy. Prior to discharge, the nurse anticipates the following antibiotics to be switched and be given orally. Select all that apply:

A) Isoniazid

B) Ampicillin

C) Tobramycin

D) Vancomycin

E) Amphotericin B

Ans: A, B

Feedback:

Switching intravenous antibiotics to oral form should be done at once. Examples of antibiotics that can be switched to its oral form include Isoniazid and Ampicillin. Amphotericin B, Vancomycin and aminoglycosides such as Tobramycin are not administered orally because of their poor gastrointestinal absorption. These medications are given parenterally to maximize their serum concentrations.

2. A premature infant suddenly developed erratic respirations, distention of the abdomen, and cyanosis. The presence of "gray syndrome" is suspected. The nurse knows that this condition is most likely caused by which medication?

A) Bacitracin

B) Clindamycin

C) Polymyxin B

D) Chloramphenicol

Ans: D

Feedback:

A serious adverse effect of Chloramphenicol is gray syndrome. This condition is manifested by cyanosis, distention of the abdomen, irregular or erratic respirations, collapse of the blood vessels, and death. The other options are incorrect.

3. A patient who recently underwent a kidney transplant is taking Cyclosporine. Which of the following statements made by the patient indicate a need for further teaching?

A) "I will stay away from patients who have active infection."

B) "I should have my kidney function be monitored closely."

C) "I don't take any other medications for pain except for Ibuprofen"

D) "I will check with my physician first before I take any antibiotic."

Ans: C

Feedback:

Cyclosporine causes immunosuppression. Hence, the patient should avoid being in contact with persons who have active infection (Option A). This medication may also lead to nephrotoxicity in large doses. Therefore, kidney function should be monitored closely (Option B). Cyclosporine should not be administered with medications that can also cause nephrotoxicity such as aminoglycosides (Option D) and non-steroidal anti-inflammatory drugs such as Ibuprofen.

4. A 5-year-old child was admitted because of aspirin poisoning. The mother suspects that her daughter has ingested the medication over an hour ago and she is very apprehensive. Upon assessment, the nurse expects to note the following signs. Select all that apply:

A) Dyspnea

B) Bleeding

C) Jaundice

D) Rapid pulse

E) Clammy extremities

Ans: A, D, E

Feedback:

Acute aspirin poisoning usually presents with difficulty of breathing, rapid pulse, and cold and clammy extremities. Bleeding and jaundice are signs of chronic aspirin overdose.

5. A patient with a history of bipolar disorder has been brought to the emergency department because of chronic constipation. She states she tried to manage the problem by taking psyllium. History taking revealed that the patient has been prescribed Lithium to help control mania. Based on the nurse's assessment, the appropriate nursing intervention would be to:

A) Document the assessment

B) Refer the patient to a psychiatrist

C) Explain that psyllium blocks the absorption of Lithium

D) Explain that psyllium potentiates the effect of Lithium; thus may increase the risk for toxicity

Ans: C

Feedback:

Psyllium is a bulk-forming laxative that is used to manage constipation and to decrease cholesterol levels. Psyllium should not be taken together with Lithium because it blocks the absorption of the medication (Lithium) leading to a decrease in the therapeutic effectiveness of the drug.

6. The nurse is caring for a patient infected with Clostridium difficile. Which of the following medications does the nurse anticipate to be prescribed?

A) Linezolid

B) Daptomycin

C) Fidaxomicin

D) Tigecycline

Ans: C

Feedback:

Fidaxomicin is a new drug approved for the treatment of Clostridium difficile infections. Its effects are concentrated in the gastrointestinal tract and there is a minimal systemic absorption. Linezolid, Daptomycin and Tigecycline are used to treat infections like Vancomycin and Methicillin (VRSA and MRSA) resistant infections of the skin and other related skin structures.

7. A patient with chronic depression has been started on monoamine oxidase inhibitors (MAOIs). The nurse discussed the need to avoid the intake of tyramine-containing foods. Teaching has been effective if the patient verbalizes to avoid the following. Select all that apply.

A) Pork

B) Soy sauce

C) Apple

D) Ripe avocado

E) Blue cheddar cheese

Ans: B, D, E

Feedback:

Monoamine oxidase inhibitors should not be taken with tyramine-rich foods because of the risk of hypertension, which may lead to hypertensive crisis. Examples of tyramine containing foods are soy sauce, ripe fruits and aged cheese.

8. A 47-year-old male client with chronic alcoholism has been prescribed to take disulfiram (Antabuse). In the administration of this medication, the nurse anticipates to perform these interventions. Select all that apply.

A) Let the patient wear a medical information identification

B) Do not let the patient know that the drug is being administered

C) Treatment should begin at least 24 hours after drinking alcohol

D) Explain that the medication may start to take effect after 12 hours

E) Instruct the patient to avoid any other forms of alcohol except medications

Ans: A, D

Feedback:

Disulfiram (Antabuse) is a drug used to treat long standing alcoholism. Nursing considerations in the administration of this medication include:

- Letting the patient wear a medical information identification
- Always alerting the patient that the drug is being administered
- Beginning the treatment at least 12 hours after drinking alcohol
- Explaining that the medication may start to take effect after 12 hours
- Instructing the patient to avoid any other forms of alcohol including Alcohol-containing medications

9. A 4-month-old infant with meningitis is receiving meropenem (Merrem IV). Due to the nature of this drug, nursing assessment should focus on which bodily system?

A) circulatory

B) respiratory

C) genitourinary

D) gastrointestinal

Ans: D

Feedback:

Meropenem is an intravenous antibiotic used in treating intraabdominal infections and meningitis. The most serious and common adverse effect of this medication involves the gastrointestinal system. Pseudomembranous colitis has been linked to the use of meropenem.

10. Lory, an 18-year-old female has been prescribed to take penicillin V (Veetids) 250 mg three times a day for a week for the treatment of urinary tract infection. The nurse instructs Lory to take the medication:

A) With meals

B) With fruit juice

C) 2-3 hours after meals

D) 30 minutes before meals

Ans: C

Feedback:

Penicillins are best absorbed on an empty stomach, usually an hour before or 2-3 hours after meals. The medication should be taken with a full 8-oz glass of water. To maximize the efficacy of the drug, it should not be taken with fruit juices, milk or soda.

11. A patient who was recently diagnosed with tuberculosis has been prescribed isoniazid (INH), rifampin (Rifadin) and pyridoxine (Vitamin B6). The client says, "I know I have to take the antibiotics for my infection but what is the Vitamin B6 for? This is the first time I have taken too many drugs." The nurse correctly responds by saying:

A) "The physician may have made a mistake. I will verify the order for Vitamin B6."

B) "Neuropathy is associated with the use of isoniazid. Pyridoxine or Vitamin B6 helps prevent this side effect."

C) "Vitamin B6 reverses the side effects of Rifampin. It is mandatory that you take all three medications"

D) "The antibiotics may lead to a decreased Vitamin B6 level. You need to take Vitamin B6 to replace the lost vitamins"

Ans: Ans: B

Feedback:

Pyridoxine (Vitamin B6) is used to counteract neuropathy, a side effect of isoniazid (INH). The other options do not support the accurate purpose of Vitamin B6

12. Docosanol (Abreva) was prescribed by a physician. The nurse knows that this medication is used to treat:

A) Genital and perianal warts

B) Canker sores

C) Cytomegalovirus for patients with AIDS

D) Oral and facial herpes simplex cold sores

Ans: D

Feedback:

Docosano (Abreva) is an antiviral medication used for treating fever blisters and cold sores in the mouth and face caused by the herpes simplex virus (herpes labialis). The other options are incorrect.

13. The nurse is caring for Tony, a 25-year-old male with histoplasmosis. Ketoconazole (Nizoral) has been prescribed. Which of the following should the nurse monitor because of potential side effects:

A) Liver enzymes

B) Hearing acuity

C) Deep tendon reflexes

D) Complete blood count

Ans: A

Feedback:

Ketoconazole has been related to severe hepatic toxicity. Hence, close monitoring of the client's liver function is necessary.

14. The nurse working in a pediatric ward receives a telephone order from the physician for an 8-year-old weighing 28 kg. The physician ordered clindamycin (Cleocin) 250 mg PO TID for 7 days. The therapeutic dose range is 8-25 mg/kg/day. What is the best nursing action?

A) Ask another nurse to verify if the order is correct

B) Contact the pharmacist to recalculate the dosage.

C) Give the medication because it is within the therapeutic dose range

D) Call the physician and clarify the order because the ordered dose is out of the therapeutic dose range

Ans: D

Feedback:

The therapeutic dose range is 8-25 mg/kg/day.

Ordered dose: 250 mg x 3 = 750 mg/day

Highest safe dose: 25 mg X 28 kg = 700 mg/ day

Lowest safe dose: 8 mg X 28 kg = 224 mg/day

- The ordered dose is 50 mg higher than the therapeutic dose. The nurse should call the physician to verify the order.

15. A post-stroke patient is about to be discharged on warfarin therapy. Which of the following herbal medications and supplements the patient is currently taking should the nurse be most concerned about? Select all that apply.

A) Ginger

B) Garlic

C) Vitamin D

D) Vitamin B12

E) Gingko biloba

Ans: A, B, E

Feedback:

Ginger, garlic and gingko biloba alter platelet aggregation increasing the risk of bleeding for patients on warfarin therapy. Supplements suspected to have the same effect include Vitamins A, C and E.

16. The physician ordered the administration of clindamycin and gentamicin to be given via intravenous piggyback (IVPB) in the same hour every 8 hours (7-3-11). How would the nurse administer the drugs?

A) Administer both drugs together via intravenous push.

B) Administer both drugs separately, flushing in between medications.

C) Administer clindamycin every 6 hours and gentamicin every 8 hours.

D) Administer one drug first, wait for an hour, and then administer the other drug.

Ans: B

Feedback:

Antibiotics should be administered one at a time; hence, if medications are ordered to be given at the same hour, the nurse needs to flush the tubing between administrations. Medications should be administered at the prescribed time.

17. The nurse is preparing to administer a bitter-tasting medication to a 1 ½ -year-old toddler. Which of the following nursing actions is appropriate?

A) Mix the medication with the child's favorite food

B) Combine the medication with orange juice to mask the taste

C) Administer the medication using a dropper at the back of the child's tongue.

D) Use an oral syringe and administer the medication between the gum and the cheek.

Ans: D

Feedback:

In administering medications to young children, the syringe is placed at the side of the mouth or between the gum and the cheek to prevent aspiration of the medication. Administering the medication at the back of the tongue may increase the risk for aspiration. Unpleasant tasting medications should not be mixed with food or drinks because the child may refuse the food or drink in the future.

18. A 30-year-old male client is about to undergo conscious sedation. The physician plans to use midazolam (Versed) for the procedure. The nurse should make sure that this medication is readily available:

A) protamine sulfate

B) naloxone (Narcan)

C) flumazenil (Romazicon)

D) phentolamine (Regitine)

Ans: C

Feedback:

Flumazenil (Romazicon) is the antidote for benzodiazepines such as Versed. Its main action is to block the action of benzodiazepine receptors. Naloxone is the antidote for narcotics; protamine sulfate for heparin and phentolamine for dopamine.

19. A 50-year-old client has been diagnosed with primary hypertension and was started on anti-hypertensive medications a week ago. The patient came back to the clinic with complaints of persistent cough. Which of the following medications is the most likely reason for the symptom the client is experiencing?

A) Hydrochlorothiazide

B) enalapril (Vasotec)

C) indapamide (Lozol)

D) amlodipine (Norvasc)

Ans: B

Feedback:

One of the side effects of angiotensin-converting enzyme inhibitors is persistent, hacking cough. The occurrence of the symptom is due to an increased sensitivity of the cough reflex. Enalapril (Vasotec) is an ACE inhibitor. hydrochlorothiazide, indapamide (thiazide diuretic) and amlodipine (calcium channel blocker) do not have cough as their side effect.

20. A patient has been receiving tolvaptan (Samsca). What should the nurse assess to check if the client is experiencing the therapeutic effect of the drug?

A) Apical pulse

B) Sodium level

C) Lipid profile

D) White blood cell count

Ans: B

Feedback:

Tolvaptan (Samsca) is a vasopressin blocker used to treat hyponatremia that cannot be treated with fluid restriction. To check the desired effect of the medication, the sodium level should be closely monitored. The other options are not directly affected by the drug.

21. Digoxin (Lanoxin) 0.125 mg PO is administered daily for a client with left ventricular heart failure. Which of the following desired changes does the nurse anticipate with the use of this drug? Select all that apply.

A) Bradypnea

B) Tachycardia

C) Decreased edema

D) Increase in urine output

E) Diminished heart murmur

Ans: C, D

Feedback:

Digoxin (Lanoxin) is a cardiac glycoside which increases myocardial contraction, cardiac output and renal perfusion. Hence, the desired effects of the drug include decreased edema and increase in urine output. Digoxin does not affect heart murmur and is not directly result to bradypnea. Bradycardia, instead of tachycardia, is the expected effect of the medication.

22. The nurse is conducting an assessment on a patient with a diagnosis of premature ventricular contractions who is receiving acebutolol (Sectral) 400 mg PO twice a day. Which assessment data signifies an adverse effect of the medication?

A) Cough

B) Dysphagia

C) Xerostomia

D) Palpitations

Ans: D

Feedback:

Acebutolol is a beta-adrenergic blocking agent. Palpitations, decreased heart rate, heartbeat irregularities, difficulty breathing, signs of heart failure and unusual tiredness are some of the adverse effects. Options A, B and C are not adverse effects of this medication.

23. Bumetanide has been indicated for a hypertensive patient. What laboratory value would alert the nurse that the client is experiencing an adverse effect of the medication?

A) Sodium level of 141 meq/L

B) Chloride level of 100 meq/L

C) Potassium level of 3.2 meq/L

D) Blood urea nitrogen (BUN) level of 21 md/dL

Ans: C

Feedback:

Bumenatide is a loop diuretic. This drug can cause extreme electrolyte depletion. A potassium level of 3.2 meq/L reflects hypokalemia, one of the adverse defects of this medication. The other options indicate values that are within the normal range.

24. A client has been on antihypertensive medication for 5 months. Which of the following data would suggest that drug tolerance has developed in this client?

A) Reduction in weight

B) Decline in blood pressure

C) Intake is less than the output

D) Steady increase in blood pressure

Ans: D

Feedback:

Long-term antihypertensive use can lead to drug tolerance as evidenced by a steady increase in blood pressure. Should this occur, the health care provider should be notified at once for the medication to be changed, discontinued or modified. Aside from the gradual increase in blood pressure, the patient is also at risk for fluid retention manifested by an increase in weight and an output lesser than fluid intake.

25. To facilitate the effectiveness of oral bisacodyl (Dulcolax), the nurse should instruct the client to take the medication:

A) In the morning

B) After a full meal

C) With a glass of milk

D) On an empty stomach

Ans: D

Feedback:

Bisacodyl (Dulolax) takes effect faster when taken on an empty stomach. If taken at bedtime, the client is expected to move his bowels in the morning. Taking the medication with meals and with a glass of milk will affect absorption.

26. The nurse is providing discharge instructions about the prescribed home medications that can cause the urine to turn orange in color. The nurse is correct when she includes these medications in the discussion. Select all that apply.

A) rifampin (Rifadin)

B) propofol (Diprivan)

C) indomethacin (Indocin)

D) sulfasalazine (Azulfidine)

E) phenazopyridine (Pyridium)

Ans: A, D, E

Feedback:

Use of rifampin, sulfasalazine and phenazopyridine can alter the urine color to orange. Propofol and indomethacin can turn the urine blue or green.

27. The nurse is reviewing the recent laboratory results of a patient on multiple medications. Which of the following laboratory values entails further follow-up? Select all that apply.

A) Digoxin level of 3 ng/ml

B) Blood sugar of 98 mg/dL

C) Sodium level of 142 meq/L

D) Lithium level of 1.8 meq/L

E) White blood cell count of 5,000 cells/ mm3

Ans: A, D

Feedback:

The therapeutic digoxin level is 0.5-2 ng/ml while for lithium, it is 0.6-1.2 meq/L. The other laboratory values are within normal limits.

28. Heparin infusion therapy has been indicated for a patient with thrombophlebitis. 24 hours after the infusion, the client's partial thromboplastin time (PTT) is noted to be 70 seconds with a control of 30 seconds. The nurse's appropriate action is to:

A) Document the findings

B) Immediately stop the infusion

C) Administer protamine sulfate

D) Report the laboratory results to the physician

Ans: A

Feedback:

The PTT indicates the effectiveness of the heparin therapy. The normal range for PTT is 60-70 seconds while on heparin therapy. The PTT is within the therapeutic range. Options B, C, and D are unnecessary.

29. A patient with myxedema coma has been prescribed to take Levothyroxine. In providing health education, the nurse plans to include these instructions. Select all that apply.

A) The medication may take several weeks to take effect

B) If stomach pain occurs, stop the medication immediately.

C) Take the medication right before lunch with a glass of water

D) Notify the physician immediately for dyspnea, fever, chills or unusual sweating.

E) While taking this medication, follow-up is necessary including blood tests to check for thyroid gland activity

Ans: A, D, E

Feedback:

Levothyroxine is a thyroid hormone. To prevent insomnia, the medication should be taken in the morning with a full glass of water. The drug should not be halted immediately because of the risk of serious effects. Should there be any dyspnea, fever, chills or unusual sweating, the physician should be notified immediately. The patient should also be reminded that the medication takes effect usually between 1-3 weeks and that follow-up is necessary to check for thyroid gland activity.

30. A patient is being discharged to home with sublingual nitroglycerin to be taken as needed for angina. Which of the following statements made by the patient signifies that the patient understood the instructions?

A) "I can use additional tablets every 3 minutes as needed"

B) "I may experience severe headaches with this medication"

C) "I occasionally use Viagra to relish some time with my wife"

D) "After taking nitroglycerin, I should wait 30 minutes before I can take my anti-hypertensive medication."

Ans: B

Feedback:

Nitroglycerin is a nitrate whose main function is to dilate the blood vessels. Because of its vasodilatory effect, it can cause severe headaches especially when used for the first time. Nitroglycerin should not be combined with Viagra or other anti-hypertensive medications because of the risk of hypotensive crisis. Additional tablets can be used every 5 minutes as needed but no more than 3 tablets in 15 minutes.

31. A patient's potassium level is low. The physician was notified and an order for the administration of intravenous potassium was made. The drug at hand is the concentrated type in an ampule. What is the appropriate action of the nurse?

A) Do not administer with Glucose 4% solution

B) Make sure to dilute the medication as directed.

C) Administer the medication via intravenous (IV) push.

D) Run the medication using a filter in the intravenous line.

Ans: B

Feedback:

Potassium irritates the vein and can cause phlebitis if not diluted. The medication should be administered via an IV pump and should never be given as a bolus. An IV filter is not necessary. The medication can be given using peripheral intravenous line. A central catheter is not mandatory.

32. A pregnant patient with severe preeclampsia is taking magnesium sulfate. Which of the following nursing interventions is appropriate?

A) Schedule a biophysical profile daily

B) Perform a non-stress test every 8 hours

C) Monitor for signs and symptoms of labor

D) Assess for signs and symptoms of infection

Ans: C

Feedback:

Magnesium sulfate is a central nervous system depressant and anticonvulsant. Having sedation as one of its effect, the patient may not be able to perceive that she is already in labor. Hence, she should be monitored for signs and symptoms of labor. Although patients with severe preeclampsia who are taking magnesium sulfate need to be monitored closely, biophysical profile and non-stress test may be done but not as frequent as what was stated in the options. Infection is usually not associated with magnesium sulfate use.

33. A patient on chemotherapy has been ordered to take epoetin alfa (Procrit). Which of the following supplements should the nurse instruct the client to strictly adhere to while taking Procrit?

A) Iron
B) Zinc
C) Vitamin E
D) Magnesium

Ans: A

Feedback:

Epoetin alfa (Procrit) is a glycoprotein very significant in the stimulation of red blood cell production or erythropoiesis. Iron is necessary for the production of red blood cells; otherwise, erythropoiesis will not be possible. The other options do not directly affect the action of Procrit.

34. A patient with epilepsy is being discharged home. Clonazepam (Klonopin) has been ordered as a home medication. The nurse instructs the patient not to abruptly cease the intake of this medication to avoid the following withdrawal symptoms. Select all that apply.

A) Tremors

B) Sweating

C) Depression

D) Increased salivation

E) Nervousness

Ans: A, B, E

Feedback:

Withdrawal symptoms can possibly occur should benzodiazepines be abruptly discontinued. These symptoms include tremors, sweating and nervousness among others. Depression and increased salivation are adverse effects of the medication.

35. The nurse is conducting an interview about the client's medication history when she came across the drug chlorthalidone (Hygroton). The nurse is aware that this medication is being taken by the client to treat which disorder?

A) Gout

B) Hypertension

C) Diabetes mellitus

D) Systemic lupus erythematosus

Ans: B

Feedback:

Chlorthalidone (Hygroton) is a thiazide-like diuretic indicated for patients with edema caused by heart failure and those with hypertension. This drug is being used with caution for patients with gout, diabetes mellitus and systemic lupus erthymatosus because of the drug's ability to alter fluid and electrolyte balance.

36. A patient has recently been prescribed with olanzapine (Zyprexa). The nurse anticipates this medication to be given in conjunction with Zyprexa:

A) Anticonvulsant

B) Antidepressant

C) Antihypertensive

D) Antiparkinsonian

Ans: D

Feedback:

Olanzapine (Zyprexa) is a dopamine antagonist. Hence, some of its side effects might include Parkinson-like side effects such as stiff muscles, twitching or uncontrolled eye movements, dry mouth or thirst. These side effects are due to the decreased dopamine in the system. To counteract this side effect, antiparkinsonian medications are usually given.

37. Tamoxifen (Soltamox) is being administered to a patient with breast cancer. Which among the following symptoms are expected to occur with this medication?

A) Nausea

B) Retinopathy

C) Pain

D) Visual acuity changes

E) Bone marrow depression

Ans: A, B, D, E

Feedback:

Tamoxifen (Soltamox) is a hormone modulator commonly used as a cancer medication. Expected side effects of this drug include gastrointestinal symptoms such as nausea, visual acuity changes, retinopathy and bone marrow depression. Pain is not anticipated with the use of this drug.

38. A patient scheduled for hemodialysis is scheduled to take his daily dose of amlodipine (Norvasc) at 3pm. He is scheduled for dialysis at 2:30pm. When should the nurse administer the amlodipine?

A) During dialysis

B) 2 hours before dialysis

C) 24 hours after the dialysis

D) After returning from dialysis

Ans: D

Feedback:

To prevent hypotension, antihypertensive medications are to be administered after the dialysis. Another reason is to prevent the medication from being removed from the bloodstream during the procedure.

39. Fluoxetine (Prozac) has been prescribed for a depressed client. 2 weeks later, she comes back to the clinic concerned that the medication is not working. What is the appropriate response of the nurse?

A) "We have to notify your physician immediately."

B) "Are you taking any other medications?"

C) "There should have been noticeable changes a week ago."

D) "The medication should start to take effect in another 7-14 days."

Ans: D

Feedback:

Fluoxetine (Prozac) is a selective serotonin reuptake inhibitor. The medication takes effect between 2-4 weeks after intake. The other options are incorrect responses.

40. A patient is taking lithium (Lithane) for the management of mania. To determine signs of early lithium toxicity, the nurse's assessment should focus on:

A) Neurologic changes

B) Circulatory problems

C) Genitourinary alterations

D) Gastrointestinal disturbances

Ans: D

Feedback:

Gastrointestinal disturbances are one of the signs of early lithium toxicity. The most common disturbances may include nausea, vomiting and diarrhea. The other options are late signs of lithium toxicity.

41. A patient is scheduled to take spironolactone (Aldactone) and amlodipine (Norvasc) at 8 am. Before the nurse can administer the medications, the patient asked if she can have a dose of calcium salt (Tums) which was ordered as needed for indigestion. What is the nurse's best action?

A) Evaluate the client's need for the antacid

B) Administer the three medications at the same time

C) Administer the amlodipine and calcium salt first, then the spironolactone 30 minutes after

D) Administer the calcium salt first, wait an hour, then administer the spironolactone and amlodipine after

Ans: A

Feedback:

Antacids inhibit the absorption of most medications. Hence, there should be at least an hour interval before or after the medication administration with this drug. Because of the diuretic nature of the spironolactone and the antihypertensive effect of amlodipine, they should be prioritized over the antacid if at all possible. Therefore, it is best that the nurse further assess the need for the antacid.

42. The nurse observes the client taking imipramine (Tofranil) for which usual side effect of this drug?

A) Diarrhea

B) Diuresis

C) Drowsiness

D) Increased salivation

Ans: C

Feedback:

Imipramine (Tofranil) is a tricyclic antidepressant with sedation, lethargy, drowsiness, sleep disturbances and fatigue as the most common side effects. Other side effects include constipation, urinary retention and dry mouth.

43. A patient has been prescribed nitroglycerin paste. The nurse noticed that acetaminophen is also ordered prior to administering the nitrate. The rationale for this order is:

A) Fever is a side effect of nitrates.

B) Nitrates usually cause headaches.

C) Acetaminophen enhances the effect of nitrates

D) Acetaminophen will help nitrates control pain

Ans: B

Feedback:

Nitrates are potent vasodilators. In most patients, it causes headaches. Acetaminophen may be given prior to nitrate administration to prevent headaches. The other options are incorrect.

44. A client has been prescribed warfarin sodium (Coumadin). The nurse provides instructions to restrict the intake of foods that are high in Vitamin K. Health teaching has been effective if the patient identifies the following as foods that are high in Vitamin K. Select all that apply.

A) Green tea

B) Kale

C) Parsley

D) Spinach

E) Guava

Ans: A, B, C, D

Feedback:

Vitamin K antagonizes the effect of warfarin sodium (Coumadin), an anti-coagulant. Green vegetables such as kale, parsley and spinach are rich in Vitamin K. Caffeine-containing beverages such as coffee and green tea are also rich in Vitamin K. Guavas are rich in Vitamin C.

45. The nurse is providing health education to a patient taking spironolactone (Aldactone). The nurse's discussion should include the following information. Select all that apply.

A) Take the medication in the morning.

B) Increase your intake of green, leafy vegetables

C) Expect that you are going to urinate more often.

D) Replace sodium in your diet using salt substitutes

E) Be sure to take the medication on an empty stomach.

Ans: A, C

Feedback:

Spironolactone (Aldactone) is a potassium-sparing diuretic. The drug should be taken in the morning and with meals. Since the drug is a diuretic, the patient should expect to urinate more often. The patient does not need to increase the intake of green, leafy vegetables since this action might further increase the potassium level in the blood. Salt substitutes usually contain potassium, hence, should also be avoided.

46. The nurse is caring for a patient with diabetes insipidus, hypotension and dehydration. Which of the following medications does the nurse anticipate to be given to this patient?

A) furosemide (Lasix)

B) glimepiride (Amaryl)

C) desmopressin (Stimate)

D) spironolactone (Aldactone)

Ans: C

Feedback:

Desmopressin is a hormone that has an antidiuretic effect. It is indicated for patients with diabetes insipidus. Furosemide and spironolactone are not to be given because of their diuretic effect. The patient is already dehydrated. Glimepiride is prescribed for type 2 diabetic patients.

47. The nurse administered 10 units of Humulin R insulin to a diabetic patient at 6 am. The nurse is aware that the patient is at most risk for hypoglycemia between:

A) 8am-10am

B) 2 pm-4pm

C) 12 noon- 2 pm

D) 10 am- 12 noon

Ans: A

Feedback:

Humulin R is short-acting insulin which starts to take effect in 30 minutes. Its peak action occurs between 2-4 hours and controls the blood sugar for as long as 6 hours. Hypoglycemia usually occurs during its peak action. In this case, the peak action is between 8am-10am.

48. The nurse is preparing to administer otic drops to a 2-year-old child. Which of the following nursing actions is correct?

A) Pull the pinna up and back and direct the solution into the ear canal

B) Pull the pinna down and back and direct the solution into the ear drum

C) Pull the auricle up and back and direct the solution into the wall of the ear canal

D) Pull the auricle down and back and direct the solution into the wall of the ear canal

Ans: D

Feedback:

To straighten the auditory canal of children 3 years old and below, the pinna or auricle must be pulled down and back. The medication is then directed to the wall of the ear canal instead of administering the medication directly to the ear drum. The other options are incorrect.

49. Valproic acid (Depakene) has been prescribed to be given once a day for a patient with a history of seizures. When is the best time to administer the medication to enhance safety?

A) At bedtime
B) After lunch
C) Before dinner
D) Before breakfast

Ans: A

Feedback:

Central nervous system depression is one of the side effects of valproic acid (Depakene), an anticonvulsant. Signs of CNS depression include sedation and dizziness. When administered at bedtime, the risk for injury secondary to its sedative effect is reduced thereby enhancing client safety.

50. A patient is on anticoagulant therapy. In developing a plan of care for this client, priority nursing actions should focus on the prevention of:

A) Injury

B) Infection

C) Dehydration

D) Hallucination

Ans: A

Feedback:

Because of the inhibition of the clotting mechanisms brought about by the effects of anticoagulants, the patient is at increased risk for injury. Hemorrhage, bleeding or bruising may happen during simple activities of daily living. The other options are not directly related to anticoagulant therapy.

51. Pentamidine isethionate (Pentam 300) is due to be administered intravenously for the treatment of leishmaniasis. Prior to administering the medication, what is an essential nursing action?

A) Place on isolation precautions

B) Promote passive exercises

C) Administer anticholinergic drugs

D) Instruct to assume a supine position

Ans: D

Feedback:

Abrupt hypotension is one of the most serious adverse effects of pentamidine isethionate (Pentam 300), an anti-infective medication. To promote safety, the patient should be in a lying position during drug administration. The other options are unnecessary nursing actions for this medication.

52. Amphotericin B has been prescribed for a patient with a fungal infection. To check for the adverse effect of the medication, the nurse should closely monitor which serum electrolyte?

A) Chloride

B) Calcium

C) Potassium

D) Bicarbonate

Ans: C

Feedback:

Hypokalemia is one of the adverse effects of amphotericin B. Manifestations of hypokalemia include electrocardiogram changes and muscle weakness. The other electrolytes are not directly affected by the medication.

53. The nurse just received the recent phenytoin (Dilantin) level result of a patient which revealed 8 mcg/ml. How should the nurse interpret this value?

A) The result is inconclusive.

B) The level is below the expected therapeutic range.

C) The level is above the expected therapeutic range

D) The result is within the expected therapeutic range.

Ans: B

Feedback:

The desired therapeutic range for phenytoin (Dilantin) is 10-20 mcg/ml. The level indicated is below the therapeutic range. This puts the patient at risk for seizures; hence, the dose should be adjusted to achieve the desired therapeutic level.

54. At 6:30 am, the nurse administered 35 units of NPH insulin to a patient with a blood glucose level of 190 mg/dl. The estimated duration of the effectiveness of this medication is:

A) 6 to 8 hours

B) 8 to 12 hours

C) 12 to 16 hours

D) 16 to 24 hours

Ans: D

Feedback:

NPH is intermediate-acting insulin. It is given daily because the duration of its effect ranges from 16 to 24 hours. The other options are incorrect.

55. An intravenous bolus of lidocaine hydrochloride (Xylocaine) has been indicated for a patient with arrhythmia. Because of the side effects of this medication, what assessment parameter should the nurse monitor?

A) Lipid profile
B) Radial pulse
C) Level of consciousness
D) Serum potassium

Ans: C

Feedback:

Lidocaine hydrochloride (Xylocaine) is an antiarrhythmic medication that can cause drowsiness, confusion and paresthesias. Level of consciousness and responsiveness should be closely monitored. Lipid profile and serum potassium are not directly influenced by lidocaine. Instead of checking the radial pulse, the nurse should monitor the apical pulse.

56. The nurse caring for a client on furosemide (Lasix) should advise the patient to increase the intake of which food?

A) Apple

B) Orange

C) Guava

D) Cantaloupe

Ans: D

Feedback:

Furosemide (Lasix) is a non-potassium sparing diuretic. The loss of potassium can be replaced by the intake of cantaloupe which contains a high level of potassium. The other options may be a source of potassium but primarily, they are good sources of Vitamin C.

57. A patient is supposed to have his serum digoxin level drawn. When should the nurse anticipate the blood to be obtained?

A) Just after the drug is administered

B) At least 6 hours after the previous dose was administered

C) An hour after the drug is administered

D) 30 minutes after the drug is administered

Ans: B

Feedback:

To make certain that the digoxin level is within the therapeutic range, serum digoxin levels should be drawn before the administration of the medication at least 6 hours after the previous dose to avoid false positive results.

58. The nurse is providing instructions on the proper intake of aluminum hydroxide, magnesium hydroxide tablets. Her instructions should include:

A) Taking the tablet with a laxative

B) Swallowing the tablet whole with a glass of water

C) Chewing the tablet completely then drinking water

D) Taking the tablet 30 minutes prior to taking another medication

Ans: C

Feedback:

Aluminum hydroxide, magnesium hydroxide antacid tablets should be chewed properly. The medication should not be swallowed whole and should not be taken with a laxative. Other medications should be given at least 1 hour prior to the administration of antacids so as not to interfere with the absorption of the other drugs.

59. Benzonatate (Tessalon) has been newly prescribed for a client. The patient asks the nurse what the medication is for. The nurse accurately responds by saying the medication:

A) Decreases anxiety

B) Promotes comfort

C) Enhances breathing

D) Treats non-productive cough

Ans: D

Feedback:

Benzonatate (Tessalon) is an antitussive used to calm persistent, non-productive cough. The other options are not the intended effects of benzonatate.

60. A patient has been ordered to take prednisone. The nurse became concerned after having reviewed the patient's medication administration record when she noticed that the patient is concurrently on this medication.

A) ibuprofen (Motrin)

B) guaifenesin

C) Cephalexin (Keflex)

D) acetaminophen (Tylenol)

Ans: A

Feedback:

Prednisone is a gastrointestinal irritant. The intake of ibuprofen (Motrin), an NSAID, can further aggravate the risk for irritation of the gastrointestinal mucosa. Hence, the use of corticosteroids and non-steroidal anti-inflammatory drugs concurrently is not recommended. The other medications do not pose a threat to the concurrent use if prednisone.

61. Methylergonovine (Methergine) is ordered to be given to a postpartum mother who just delivered a healthy newborn. Prior to administering the medication, what is the nurse's priority nursing action to establish baseline data in the assessment of possible side effects?

A) Assess temperature

B) Check the blood pressure

C) Perform a neurologic assessment

D) Monitor respiratory rate

Ans: B

Feedback:

Methylergonovine (Methergine) is an oxytocic agent used to promote uterine involution. One of its serious side effects is the elevation of blood pressure. Hence, the blood pressure should always be checked prior to the administration of the medication. The other options are usual assessment procedures following delivery.

62. A patient with acute leukemia is taking mercaptopurine (Purinethol). The nurse should make sure that the client is adequately hydrated because of the increased chances of:

A) dehydration

B) hypotension

C) hyperuricemia

D) hypernatremia

Ans: C

Feedback:

Mercaptopurine (Purinethol) is an antimetabolite used in the treatment of acute leukemia. Usual concerns with the use of this drug include bone marrow depression and gastrointestinal disturbances. A concerning side effect is hyperuricemia. To prevent further complications, the nurse has to make sure that the patient is adequately hydrated.

63. The nurse is caring for a patient with a history of simple partial seizures. Which of the following medications will most likely be prescribed as an adjunct therapy medication?

A) Diazepam (Valium)

B) Gabapentin (Neurontin)

C) Phenobarbital (Luminal)

D) Phensuximide (Milontin)

Ans: B

Feedback:

Gabapentin (Neurontin) is an anticonvulsant indicated for the treatment of partial seizures. Diazepam (Valium) and phenobarbital (Luminal) are usually indicated for status epilepticus while phensuximide (Milontin) usually treats absence seizure disorder.

64. A patient with Zollinger-Ellison syndrome reports the presence of headache. Which of the following medications can be safely administered?

A) Ibuprofen (Advil)

B) Ketoprofen (Actron)

C) Acetaminophen (Tylenol)

D) Acetylsalicylic acid (Aspirin)

Ans: C

Feedback:

Zollinger-Ellison syndrome is characterized by an overproduction of gastric acid in the stomach. Among the given options, acetaminophen (Tylenol) is the only safe medication to be administered. Acetylsalicylic acid (Aspirin) and non-steroidal anti-inflammatory drugs such as ketoprofen and ibuprofen are gastric irritants and should not be administered to patients with Zollinger-Ellison syndrome.

65. An 8-year-old child with attention deficit hyperactivity disorder has been prescribed methylphenidate (Concerta) tablets 5 mg orally twice daily. The nurse instructs the mother to administer the medication at which times?

A) Before lunch and before dinner

B) With breakfast and with dinner

C) With lunch and before bedtime

D) Before breakfast and before lunch

Ans: D

Feedback:

Methylphenidate (Concerta) is a central nervous system stimulant. Twice a day dosing should be taken before breakfast and before lunch. The medication should not be administered in the afternoon or in the evening because the drug can cause insomnia secondary to its stimulating effect.

66. Propantheline has been indicated for a patient with peptic ulcer disease. Teaching has been effective regarding the use of this drug when the patient states:

A) "I should take this medication with meals."

B) "I am going to take this medication just after meals."

C) "This medication works best when taken with antacids."

D) "I should take this medication 30 minutes before meals."

Ans: D

Feedback:

Propantheline is an anticholinergic/ parasympatholytic agent. Its main function includes decreasing gastrointestinal secretions and spasms. Because of the nature of the medication, it has to be administered 30 minutes before meals. The other options are incorrect.

67. A patient on carbamazepine (Tegretol) for the treatment of tonic-clonic seizure has been instructed to notify the health care provider immediately if which of the following symptoms are experienced?

A) Fever

B) Nausea

C) Vomiting

D) Dizziness

Ans: A

Feedback:

Patients taking carbamazepine (Tegretol) should be closely monitored for blood dyscrasia, an adverse effect of the drug. Signs of blood dyscrasia include fever, mouth sores, sore throat and unusual bleeding among others. Options B, C and D are usual side effects of the medication.

68. The nurse caring for a patient on donepezil hydrochloride (Aricept) has her care plan focused on addressing which medical condition?

A) Dementia

B) Depression

C) Schizophrenia

D) Panic disorder

Ans: A

Feedback:

Donepezil (Aricept) is used in managing Alzheimer's dementia. It is a cholinergic agent used to elevate acetylcholine levels; hence, aids in slowing down the progression of the disease. Donepezil is not indicated for the other medical conditions.

69. The nurse caring for a patient with major depressive disorder is taking escitalporam (Lexapro). After a thorough review of the client's medical history, the nurse puts the medication on hold and calls the physician immediately if which assessment data is noted?

A) A history of diabetes mellitus

B) Use of Cephalexin (Keflex)

C) Use of isocarboxacid (Marplan)

D) A history of barrier contraceptive use

Ans: C

Feedback:

Escitalopram (Lexapro) is a serotonin reuptake inhibitor. To avoid the risk of complications from serotonin syndrome, the medication should not be combined with a monoamine oxidase inhibitor (isocarboxacid). Otherwise, the concurrent use of both drugs can be fatal..

70. A patient who had a minor vehicular accident has been prescribed to take carisoprodol (Soma). Which of the following assessment data would signify a desired effect of the medication?

A) Controlled bleeding

B) Resolved infection

C) Decreased muscle spasms

D) Decrease in blood pressure

Ans: C

Feedback:

Carisorpodol (Soma) is a centrally acting skeletal muscle relaxant. It is used primarily to relieve muscle pain and discomfort. The other options are not the intended effect of the medication.

71. A patient has been ordered to take risperidone (Risperdal) for bipolar disorder. Which laboratory test should the nurse initially check before administering the medication?

A) Magnesium levels

B) Coagulation studies

C) Liver function tests

D) Complete blood count

Ans: C

Feedback:

Risperidone (Risperdal) is an antipsychotic medication which acts to control behavioral responses. Prior to giving the drug, renal and liver function tests should be initiated. Patients with renal or hepatic problems, those with cardiovascular disorders and older adults should be monitored closely if they are to use this medication.

72. Discharge instructions are being given for a patient going home on Zolpidem (Ambien). For the medication to achieve its maximum effect, the nurse instructs the client to take the drug with:

A) milk

B) dinner

C) antacid

D) a glass of water

Ans: D

Feedback:

The anxiolytic medication zolpidem (Ambien) should be taken at bedtime and should be swallowed whole with a full glass of water. The medication should not be taken with meals, milk or antacid to maximize its absorption.

73. The nurse is working in a cardiac unit and is aware that the drug of choice for the initial treatment of life-threatening ventricular dysrhythmias is:

A) Ranolazine (Ranexa)

B) Disopyramide (Norpace)

C) Amiodarone (Cordarone)

D) Isosorbide dinitrate (Isordil)

Ans: C

Feedback:

Amiodarone (Cordarone) is a class III antiarrhythmic agent used to suppress unstable ventricular tachycardia. Amiodarone is the drug of choice because it is safe and efficient even in cardiac arrests that happen out of the hospital. Disopyramide (Norpace) is also an antiarrhythmic medication but only comes in oral form. Ronalazine and isosorbide dinitrate are medications for angina.

74. A patient has been started on tissue plasminogen activator therapy (Activase). In providing care for this client, the nurse has ensure that this equipment is always on hand:

A) Scissors

B) Hemostat

C) Suction equipment

D) Occult blood test strips

Ans: D

Feedback:

Tissue plasminogen activators are thrombolytic agents. A usual side effect of these medications is bleeding. For the nurse to effectively monitor signs of bleeding, occult blood test strips should be readily available. The test strips will especially be useful in checking the presence of blood in the stool, urine or gastric drainage. The other options are not particularly helpful in monitoring bleeding.

75. A patient with Parkinson's disease is taking benztropine mesylate (Cogentin). Which of the following symptoms or signs exhibited by the patient signifies a side effect of the medication?

A) Fever

B) Mouth sores

C) Irregular heart rate

D) Overflow incontinence

Ans: D

Feedback:

Benztropine mesylate (Cogentin) is an anticholinergic medication. One of the side effects of the drug is retention of urine. Hence, the patient should be assessed for signs of urinary retention including dysuria, abdominal distention, and overflow incontinence. The other options are not related to the use of Cogentin.

76. A patient with acquired immunodeficiency syndrome (AIDS) is being given ganciclovir (Cytovene). Which of the following statements made by the patient reflects an understanding of the most frequent side effect of this drug?

A) "I will need to use an electric razor to shave."

B) "I have to take antihypertensive medications."

C) "I will take the medication on an empty stomach."

D) "I have to decrease my intake of foods high in sodium"

Ans: A

Feedback:

One of the most common side effects of ganciclovir (Cytovene) is thrombocytopenia. The patient should use electric razor when shaving to reduce the risk of injury that can result to bleeding. The medication need not be taken on an empty stomach. Options B and D are unrelated to the use of this drug.

77. A patient on antipsychotic medications suddenly developed hyperthermia, hypertension and muscle rigidity. The nurse suspects neuroleptic malignant syndrome. To treat this condition, the nurse anticipates the administration of:

A) Naloxone (Narcan)

B) Protamine sulfate

C) Dantrolene (Dantrium)

D) Phytonadione (Vitamin K)

Ans: C

Feedback:

Dantrolene (Dantrium), a skeletal muscle relaxant and bromocriptine (Parlodel), a dopaminergic agent, are used to ease the symptoms of neuroleptic malignant syndrome. Naloxone is the antidote for narcotic overdose. Protamine sulfate is the antidote for heparin phytonadione is the antidote for warfarin.

78. The nurse is demonstrating to a patient how to draw the NPH insulin from the vial. Which of the following nursing actions is accurate prior to aspirating the insulin?

A) Refrigerate the insulin vial

B) Remove the air from the vial

C) Rotate the insulin vial between the palms of hands

D) Shake the vial to even out the solution

Ans: C

Feedback:

To resuspend the insulin, it is essential for the nurse to rotate the insulin vial between the palms of hands. Shaking the vial is not recommended because it results in the formation of bubbles and foam. Removal of the air and refrigeration of the vial are not necessary.

79. A post-hemorrhoidectomy patient has been ordered a laxative to prevent straining. The nurse anticipates to administer this medication:

A) Senna (Senokot)

B) Docusate (Colace)

C) Bisacodyl (Dulcolax)

D) Magnesium sulfate (Epsom salts)

Ans: B

Feedback:

Docusate (Colace) is a stool softener usually that is usually used to prevent constipation and straining. It is frequently indicated for surgical, cardiac or obstetrical patients when straining is contraindicated. Senna is a laxative used for short-term relief of constipation while magnesium sulfate is used for evacuating the gastrointestinal tract quickly. Bisacodyl (Dulcolax) is a stimulant laxative drug whose desired effect is to produce a bowel movement

80. A patient is being prepared for colonoscopy. Magnesium citrate has been ordered as a bowel preparation procedure. How should the nurse administer the medication?

A) Served with ice

B) Mixed with fruit juice

C) Mixed with tepid water

D) Served cold with a full glass of water

Ans: D

Feedback:

Magnesium citrate is a saline cathartic usually used to prepare the gastrointestinal tract for diagnostic procedures. Because of its unpleasant taste, it is best administered chilled with a full glass of water. It should not be served with ice nor mixed with tepid water because these actions decrease the carbonation, making the solution more distasteful.

81. A patient was started on pancrelipase (Pancrease). The nurse knows that the desired effect of this medication is:

A) Relief from constipation

B) Relief from abdominal pain

C) Regulation of blood glucose

D) Reduction of fat in the stools

Ans: D

Feedback:

Pancrelipase (Pancrease) is used to replace inadequate pancreatic enzymes. This drug helps digest and absorb carbohydrates, proteins and fats. Its advantage includes the reduction of fat in the stools. The drug is not used to treat constipation and abdominal pain. Insulin regulates blood glucose.

82. A patient with myasthenia gravis has been prescribed pyridostigmine bromide (Mestinon). The nurse safely administers the medication by:

A) Asking the client to assume a side-lying position

B) Administering the medication with small sips of water

C) Instructing the client to take the medication with juice

D) Taking the patient's blood pressure prior to giving the medication

Ans: B

Feedback:

Myasthenia gravis is a medical condition affecting the muscular system including the patient's ability to swallow. To prevent aspiration, the patient's ability to take in oral substance, including medications, should be assessed first. The other options are unnecessary in administering pyridostigmine bromide.

83. A patient with Parkinson's disease has recently been started with levodopa. Which of the following parameters should be assessed prior to initiating ambulation?

A) History of fall

B) Muscle strength

C) Orthostatic vital signs

D) Deep tendon reflexes

Ans: C

Feedback:

Levodopa can cause orthostatic hypotension. The medication, coupled with Parkinson's disease, further increases the risk for orthostatic hypotension. Hence, prior to helping the client ambulate, the nurse's initial action is to assess the patient's orthostatic vital signs. Assessing muscle strength and history of fall is part of the assessment prior to ambulation, but are not the primary data needed in relation to the use of levodopa. Deep tendon reflexes may be part of routine assessment, but is not directly related to Levodopa and Parkinson's disease.

84. Buspirone (Vanspar) has been ordered for a client with anxiety disorder. The patient states that swallowing the medication is quite difficult. To help ease the problem, the nurse should:

A) Crush the tablets

B) Substitute a liquid form of the medication

C) Request the physician to change the medication

D) Cut the tablet in half then mix the medication with applesauce

Ans: A

Feedback:

Buspirone (Vanspar) is an antianxiety medication that comes in a tablet form. The medication can be crushed to ease swallowing. The medication does not come in a liquid form. Cutting the tablet in half and mixing it with applesauce is not a guarantee that the medication will be swallowed easily. Calling the physician to change the medication is a hasty decision especially since not all options have been exhausted.

85. A client has been taking metoclopramide (Reglan) for 6 months now. Which of the following assessment data alerts the nurse to call the physician immediately?

A) Constipation

B) Urinary retention

C) Polycythemia

D) Uninhibited rhythmic movements of the face and extremities

Ans: D

Feedback:

Tardive dyskinesia is one of the irreversible side effects of long-term metoclopramide use. This condition is manifested by uninhibited rhythmic movements of the face and extremities.

86. A patient's intravenous theophylline is due to be discontinued and switched to a sustained-release form. When is the appropriate time to administer the initial dose of the oral medication?

A) In 4-6 hours after discontinuing the intravenous form

B) Immediately after discontinuing the intravenous form

C) After 24 hours after discontinuing the intravenous form

D) After 12 hours after discontinuing the intravenous form

Ans: B

Feedback:

A sustained-release form of the medication should be administered immediately after discontinuing the intravenous form to maintain the therapeutic level of the medication. An immediate-release form of the medication, on the other hand, should be administered 4-6 hours after discontinuing the intravenous form.

87. A client with spinal problems is taking baclofen (Lioresal) for painful muscle spasms. The nurse should monitor the client for which frequent side effect of the medication?

A) Cough

B) Hypoglycemia

C) Drowsiness

D) hypertension

Ans: C

Feedback:

Baclofen (Lioresal) is a centrally acting muscle relaxant. One of its usual side effects is sedation as evidenced by drowsiness. The other symptoms are not related to baclofen use.

88. A patient on phenytoin (Dilantin) recently manifested nystagmus. How should the nurse interpret this finding?

A) The symptom is unrelated to phenytoin use.

B) Nystagmus is a side effect of the medication.

C) The phenytoin level is above the therapeutic level

D) The phenytoin level is below the therapeutic level

Ans: C

Feedback:

The presence of nystagmus signifies a phenytoin serum amount that is above the therapeutic level. The desired therapeutic level for phenytoin is 10-20 mcg/ml. Because of the presence of nystagmus, the patient's serum phenytoin level should be assessed immediately.

89. A patient with Kaposi sarcoma secondary to advanced HIV infection is taking daunorubucin (DaunoXome). The nurse should watch out for which common side effect of this medication?

A) Nystagmus

B) Hematemesis

C) Petechiae

D) Back pain

Ans: D

Feedback:

Common side effects associated with the use of daunorubicin include cough, hoarseness, dysuria, dyspnea, lower back or side pain and paresthesia.

90. A patient who recently underwent an eye surgery is due to take an ophthalmic antibiotic and a mydriatic at the same time. How should the nurse administer the ophthalmic medications?

A) Administer the medications at the same time.

B) Administer the mydriatic medication first, immediately followed by the antibiotic

C) Administer the mydriatic medication first, wait for 3 minutes, then administer the antibiotic

D) Administer the antbiotic medication first, wait for at least 15 minutes, then administer the mydriatic

Ans: C

Feedback:

If two ophthalmic medications are to be administered at the same time, the nurse should administer the medications separately with a 3-5 minute interval in between. The interval between medications is necessary to facilitate the absorption of the medications and at the same time, to prevent the second medication from cleansing out the first medication. The other options are incorrect.

91. A patient is on mitomycin (Mutamycin) for the treatment of pancreatic cancer. Which common adverse effect of mitomycin should the nurse report to the physician? Signs and symptoms of:

A) Drug induced meningitis

B) Bone marrow suppression

C) Drowsiness

D) Cardiac dysrhythmias

Ans: B

Feedback:

Patients on mitomycin (Mutamycin) should be closely monitored for signs of bone marrow toxicity such as thrombocytopenia and leukopenia.

92. The nurse is providing discharge instructions to a client going home on rifampin (Rifadin). Which of the following statements made by the patient reflect an understanding of the characteristics of the medication?

A) "My skin might temporarily be jaundiced in color."

B) "I can stop the medication once the cultures are negative."

C) "I am going to wear glasses instead of the usual contact lens."

D) "I should always take the medication 2 hours before or after meals."

Ans: C

Feedback:

Rifampin (rifadin) can cause orange discoloration of body fluids. The patient is advised to wear glasses instead of contact lenses because it can discolor the latter. Changes in skin color such as yellowish discoloration (jaundice) indicates and adverse effect of the drug. The drug may still need to be continued even if cultures are negative. If the patient experiences gastrointestinal discomfort when the drug is taken on an empty stomach, the patient may take the medication with food.

93. A patient is on intravenous vincristine (Oncovin) for the treatment of acute leukemia. Which of the following medications should be prepared if extravasation occurs?

A) Ascorbic acid

B) Hyaluronidase

C) Sodium bicarbonate

D) Isotonic sodium thiosulfate

Ans: B

Feedback:

The antidote for vincristine (Oncovin) extravasation is hyaluronidase (Wydase). The drug is administered subcutaneously. After administration of the antidote, warm compress is applied to the area to diffuse the drug and promote comfort.

94. An adolescent has been suffering from a nonproductive cough for almost a week now. The physician prescribed dextromethorphan (Benylin) to suppress the cough reflex. The nurse withholds the administration of the drug if the patient is also taking:

A) Metoprolol (Lopressor)

B) Rifampicin (Rifadin)

C) Gentamicin (Garamycin)

D) Isocarboxazid (Marplan)

Ans: D

Feedback:

Dextromethorphan should not be used concurrently with monoamine oxidase inhibitors such as Isocarboxazid (Marplan) because of the risk of the development of high blood pressure, hyperthermia, nausea, myoclonic jerks and coma. There are no contraindications to the use of dextromethorphan with the other medications presented.

95. The nurse is teaching a client how to self-administer an intranasal corticosteroid. Which of the following actions demonstrate a correct technique in the administration of the medication?

A) Sit upright with the head tilted slightly forward.

B) Place the tip of the applicator ½ inch away from the nostril

C) Press the canister halfway twice to deliver the medication

D) Vigorously breathe while spraying the medication

Ans: A

Feedback:

In administering a nasal aerosol, the patient's head should be positioned upright with the head tilted slightly forward. The applicator tip should be placed inside the nostril. Inhaling vigorously after spraying is discouraged because it delivers the medicine deep into the throat and not in the nose as intended.

96. Urokinase (Abbokinase) has been prescribed to a client with coronary thrombosis. The nurse is aware that the primary purpose of this medication is to:

A) Break down the clot

B) Prevent further clot formation

C) Decrease the formation of platelets

D) Reduce the myocardium's need for oxygen

Ans: A

Feedback:

Urokinase (Abbokinase) is a thrombolytic agent whose primary purpose is to break down the clot or thrombus. Anticoagulants prevent further clot formation while antiplatelets decrease the formation of platelets. To reduce myocardial oxygen demand, the physician may order nitrates or calcium channel blockers to name a few.

97. A client weighs 176 pounds. The provider orders a heparin bolus of 85 units per kilogram and then to initiate a maintenance infusion at 20 units per kilogram per hour. The heparin infusion is 25,000 units per liter of 0.9% Sodium Chloride. What is the needed infusion rate to achieve 20 units per kilogram per hour?

A) 60 ml/hr

B) 64 ml/hr

C) 58 ml/hr

D) 62 ml/hr

Ans: B

Feedback:

Calculate the client's weight in kilograms.

176 lbs divided by 2.2 lbs= 80 kg

Calculate the heparin bolus dosage

85 units/kg multiplied by 80 kg= 6800 units

Calculate the infusion rate for the IV dosage

20 units/kg/hr multiplied by 80 kg= 1600 units/hr

Calculate rate in ml/hr and set the pump accordingly.

1,000 ml: 25,000 units= ___ ml: 1600 units

25,000 x= 1,000 (1600)

$$\frac{25{,}000\ x = 1{,}600{,}000}{25{,}000}$$

x= 64 ml/hr

98. A patient has been recently prescribed to take felodipine (Plendil) for hypertension. Which of the following fruit juices should the nurse instruct the patient to avoid?

A) Grapefruit juice

B) Apple juice

C) Orange juice

D) Cranberry juice

Ans: A

Feedback:

Patients taking calcium channel blockers should be instructed to avoid grapefruit juice. Studies have shown that the presence of grapefruit juice in the body increases the concentration of calcium channel blockers. The other options do not directly affect calcium channel blockers.

99. Midodrine (ProAmatine) has been indicated for a patient. The nurse is aware that the medication is used to treat:

A) Infection

B) Depression

C) Chronic kidney disease

D) Orthostatic hypotension

Ans: D

Feedback:

Midodrine (ProAmatine) is an alpha-specific adrenergic agent used to treat symptomatic orthostatic hypotension in adults. Midodrine does not treat infection, depression or chronic kidney disease.

100. A patient with heart failure is not responsive to digitalis, diuretics or vasodilators. What medication does the nurse anticipate the physician to prescribe for short-term treatment of the condition?

A) Digoxin (Lanoxin)

B) Furosemide (Lasix)

C) Milrinone (Primacor)

D) Hydralazine (Apresoline)

Ans: C

Feedback:

Milrinone (Primacor) is a phosphodiesterase inhibitor used as a short term treatment for heart failure in patients where digitalis, diuretics and vasodilators are ineffective. Digoxin is a digitalis. Furosemide is a diuretic and hydralazine is a vasodilator.

Made in the USA
Columbia, SC
07 February 2021